PLANT-BASED RECIPES

An Intuitive & Complete Cookbook for Beginners

Green Kitchen

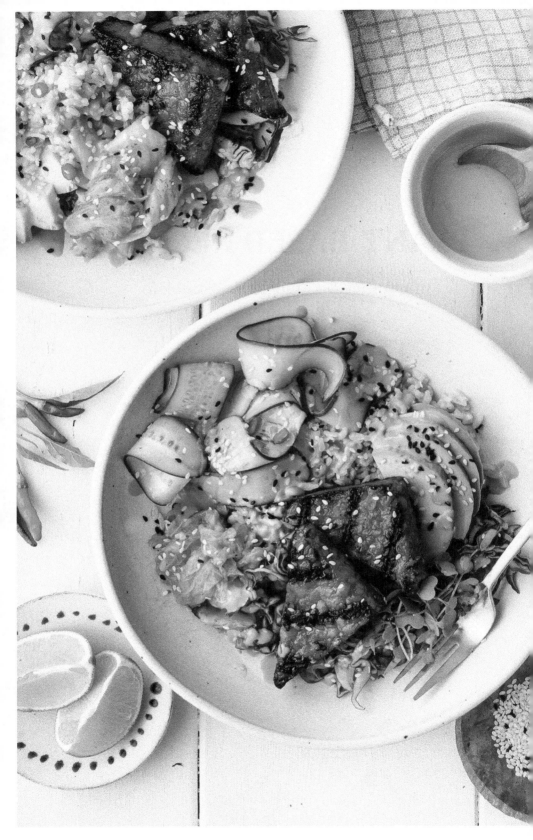

Table of Contents

BREAKFAST

Vegan Banh Mi

8 Servings

(Ready in about 35 minutes)

Nutrition: Calories: 372; Fat: 21.9g; Carbs: 29.5g; Protein: 17.6g

Ingredients

- 1 cup rice vinegar
- 1/2 cup of water
- 1/2 cup white sugar
- 4 carrots, cut into 1/16-inch-thick matchsticks
- 1 cup white (daikon) radish, cut into 1/16-inch-thick matchsticks
- 2 white onions, thinly sliced.
- 1/2 cup fresh parsley, chopped
- Kosher salt and ground black pepper, to taste
- 4 standard French baguettes, cut into four pieces
- 8 tablespoons fresh cilantro, chopped
- 8 lime wedges
- 4 tablespoons olive oil
- 24 ounces firm tofu, cut into sticks
- 1/2 cup vegan mayonnaise
- 3 tablespoons soy sauce
- 4 cloves of garlic, minced

Directions

1. Combine the rice vinegar, water, and sugar to a boil, and stir until the sugar has dissolved for about 1 minute. Allow it to cool.
2. Pour the cooled vinegar mixture over the carrot, daikon radish, and onion; allow the vegetables to marinate for at least 30 minutes.
3. While the vegetables are marinating, heat the olive oil in a frying pan over medium-high heat. Once hot, add the tofu and sauté for 8 minutes, occasionally stirring to promote even cooking.
4. Then, mix the mayo, soy sauce, garlic, parsley, salt, and ground black pepper in a small bowl.
5. Slice each piece of the baguette in half the long way. Then, toast the baguette halves under the preheated broiler for about 3 minutes.
6. To assemble the banh mi sandwiches, spread each half of the toasted baguette with the mayonnaise mixture; fill the cavity of the bottom half of the bread with the fried tofu sticks, marinated vegetables, and cilantro leaves.
7. Lastly, squeeze the lime wedges over the filling and top with the other half of the baguette.
   Bon Appetite.

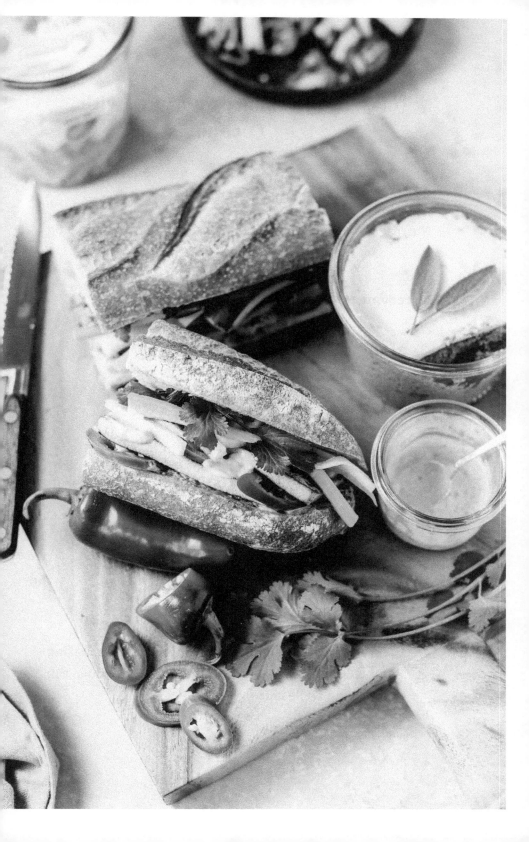

Classic Applesauce Pancakes with Coconut

16 Servings

(Ready in about 50 minutes)

Nutrition: Calories: 208; Fat: 8g; Carbs: 33.2g; Protein: 3.6g

Ingredients

- 2 1/2 cups whole-wheat flour
- 2 teaspoons baking powder
- 1/2 teaspoon sea salt
- 1 teaspoon coconut sugar
- 1/2 teaspoon ground cloves
- 1/2 teaspoon ground cardamom
- 1 teaspoon ground cinnamon
- 3/2 cup oat milk
- 1 cup applesauce, unsweetened
- 4 tablespoons coconut oil
- 16 tablespoons coconut, shredded
- 16 tablespoons pure maple syrup

Directions

1. In a mixing bowl, properly combine the flour, baking powder, salt, sugar, and spices. Gradually add in the milk and applesauce.

2. Heat a frying pan over a moderately high flame and add a small amount of coconut oil.
3. Once hot, pour the batter into the frying pan. Cook for approximately 3 minutes until the bubbles form; flip it and cook on the other side for 3 minutes longer until browned on the underside. Repeat with the remaining oil and batter.
4. Serve with shredded coconut and maple syrup. Bon appétit!

Everyday Oats with Coconut and Strawberries

4 Servings

(Ready in about 15 minutes)

Nutrition: Calories: 457; Fat: 14.4g; Carbs: 66.3g; Protein: 17.3g

Ingredients

- 1 tablespoon coconut oil
- 2 cups of rolled oats
- A pinch of flaky sea salt
- 1/4 teaspoon grated nutmeg
- 1/2 teaspoon cardamom
- 2 tablespoons coconut sugar
- 2 cups coconut milk, sweetened
- 2 cups of water
- 4 tablespoons coconut flakes
- 8 tablespoons fresh strawberries

Directions

1. In a saucepan, melt the coconut oil over a medium flame. Then, toast the oats for about 3 minutes, stirring continuously.

2. Add in the salt, nutmeg, cardamom, coconut sugar, milk, and water; continue to cook for 12 minutes more or until cooked through.
3. Spoon the mixture into serving bowls; top with coconut flakes and fresh strawberries.
   Enjoy!

Classic Applesauce Pancakes with Coconut

16 Servings

(Ready in about 60 minutes)

Nutrition: Calories: 208; Fat: 8g; Carbs: 33.2g; Protein: 3.6g

Ingredients

- 2 ½ cups whole-wheat flour
- 2 teaspoons baking powder
- 1/2 teaspoon sea salt
- 1 teaspoon coconut sugar
- 1/2 teaspoon ground cloves
- 1/2 teaspoon ground cardamom
- 1 teaspoon ground cinnamon
- 3/2 cup oat milk
- 1 cup applesauce, unsweetened
- 4 tablespoons coconut oil
- 16 tablespoons coconut, shredded
- 16 tablespoons pure maple syrup

Directions

1. Thoroughly combine the flour, baking powder, salt, sugar, and spices. Gradually add the milk and applesauce in a mixing bowl.

2. Heat a frying pan over a moderately high flame and add a small amount of coconut oil.
3. Once hot, pour the batter into the frying pan. Cook for approximately 3 minutes until the bubbles form; flip it and cook on the other side for 3 minutes longer until browned on the underside. Repeat with the remaining oil and batter.
4. Serve with shredded coconut and maple syrup. Bon appétit!

Zucchini Pancakes

8 Servings

Preparation Time: 10 minutes | **Cooking Time:** 15 minutes

Nutrition: Calories 65, Total Fat 4.7g, Saturated Fat 0.9g, Cholesterol 41mg, Sodium 97mg, Total Carbohydrate 4.1g, Dietary Fiber 0.8g, Total Sugars 1.4g, Protein 2.3g, Calcium 16mg, Iron 1mg, Potassium 175mg, Phosphorus 24mg

Ingredients:

- 4 cups zucchini
- 1/2 cup onion
- 2 tablespoons all-purpose white flour
- 2 teaspoons herb seasoning
- 2 eggs, 1 tablespoon olive oil
- 1/4 teaspoon salt

Directions:

1. Grate onion and zucchini into a bowl and stir to combine. Place the zucchini mixture on a clean kitchen towel. Twist and squeeze out as much liquid as possible. Return to the bowl.
2. Mix flour, salt, and herb seasoning in a small bowl. Add egg and mix; stir into zucchini and onion mixture. Form 4 patties.

3. Heat oil over high heat in a large non-stick frying pan. Lower heat to medium and place zucchini patties into the pan. Sauté until brown, turning once.
Enjoy!

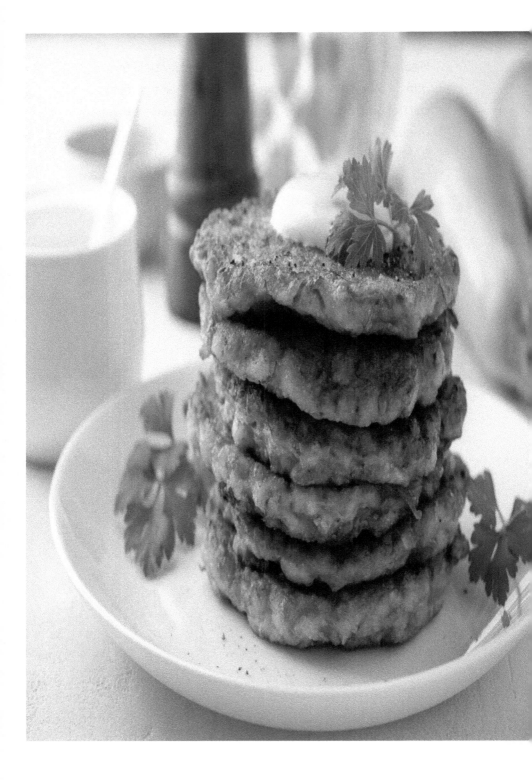

Creole Tofu Scramble

8 Servings

Preparation Time: 5-15 minutes | **Cooking Time:** 20 minutes

Nutrition: Calories 258 Fats 15. 9g Carbs 12. 8g Protein 20. 7g

Ingredients:

- 4 tbsps plant butter, for frying
- 2 (14 oz) pack firm tofu, pressed and crumbled
- 2 medium red bell peppers, deseeded and chopped
- 2 medium green bell peppers, deseeded and chopped
- 2 tomatoes, finely chopped
- 4 tbsps chopped fresh green onions
- Salt and black pepper to taste
- 2 tsps turmeric powder
- 2 tsps Creole seasoning
- 1 cup chopped baby kale
- ½ cup grated plant-based Parmesan cheese

Directions:

1. Melt the plant butter in a large skillet over medium heat and add the tofu. Cook with occasional stirring until the tofu is light golden brown while making sure not to break the tofu into tiny bits but to have scrambled egg resemblance, 5 minutes.

2. Stir in the bell peppers, tomato, green onions, salt, black pepper, turmeric powder, and Creole seasoning. Sauté until the vegetables soften, 5 minutes.
3. Mix in the kale to wilt, 3 minutes and then, half of the plant-based Parmesan cheese. Allow melting for 1 to 2 minutes, and then turn the heat off.
4. Dish the food, top with the remaining cheese, and serve warm.

   Enjoy!!

Apple Cinnamon Muffins

8 Servings

Preparation Time: 5-15 minutes | **Cooking Time:** 40 minutes

Nutrition: Calories 1133 Fats 74. 9g Carbs 104. 3g Protein 18g.

Ingredients:

For the muffins:

- 2 flax seeds powder + 3 tbsps of water
- 3 cups whole-wheat flour
- 2 1/2 cups pure date sugar
- 4 tsps baking powder
- 1/2 tsp salt
- 2 tsps cinnamon powder
- 2/3 cup melted plant butter
- 2/3 cup flax milk
- 4 apples, peeled, cored, and chopped

For topping:

- 2/3 cup whole-wheat flour
- 1 cup pure date sugar
- 1 cup cold plant butter, cubed
- 3 tsps cinnamon powder

Directions:

1. Preheat the oven to 400 F and grease 6 muffin cups with cooking spray. In a bowl, mix the flax seed powder with water and allow thickening for 5 minutes to make the flax egg.
2. In a medium bowl, mix the flour, date sugar, baking powder, salt, and cinnamon powder. Whisk in the butter, flax egg, flax milk, and then fold in the apples. Fill the muffin cups two-thirds way up with the batter.
3. In a small bowl, mix the remaining flour, date sugar, cold butter, and cinnamon powder. Sprinkle the mixture on the muffin batter. Bake for 20-minutes. Remove the muffins onto a wire rack, allow cooling, and serve warm.

Enjoy!!

Orange Granola with Hazelnuts

10 Servings

(Ready in 50 minutes)

Ingredients

- 4 cups rolled oats
- 2 1/2 cups whole-wheat flour
- 2 tbsps ground cinnamon
- 2 tsps ground ginger
- 1 cup sunflower seeds
- 1 cup hazelnuts, chopped
- 1 cup pumpkin seeds
- 1 cup shredded coconut
- 5/2 cups orange juice
- 1 cup dried cherries
- 1 cup goji berries

Directions

1. Preheat oven to 350 F.
2. In a bowl, combine the oats, flour, cinnamon, ginger, sunflower seeds, hazelnuts, pumpkin seeds, and coconut. Pour in the orange juice, toss to mix well.

3. Transfer to a baking sheet and bake for 15 minutes. Turn the granola and continue baking until it is crunchy, about 30 minutes.
4. Stir in the cherries and goji berries and store in the fridge for up to 14 days.

Enjoy!

Coconut Oat Bread

8 Servings
(Ready in 50 minutes)

Ingredients

- 8 cups whole-wheat flour
- 1/2 tsp salt
- 1 cup rolled oats
- 2 tsps baking soda
- 2 1/2 cups coconut milk, thick
- 4 tbsps pure maple syrup

Directions

1. Preheat the oven to 400 F.
2. In a bowl, mix flour, salt, oats, and baking soda.
3. Add in coconut milk and maple syrup and whisk until dough forms.
4. Dust your hands with some flour and knead the dough into a ball.
5. Shape the dough into a circle and place it on a baking sheet.
6. Cut a deep cross on the dough and bake in the oven for 15 minutes at 450 F.

7. Reduce the temperature to 400 F and bake further for 20 to 25 minutes or until a hollow sound is made when the bottom of the bread is tapped. Slice and serve.

Enjoy!

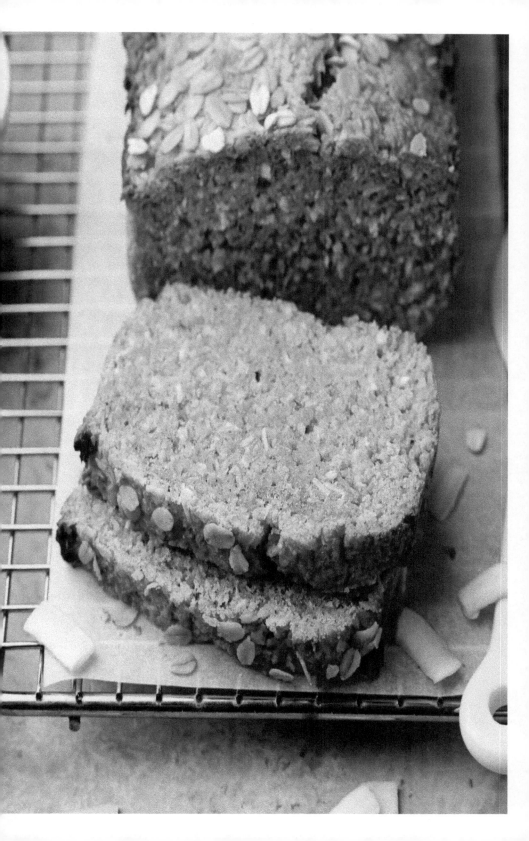

Spicy Quinoa Bowl with Black Beans

8 Servings

(Ready in 25 minutes)

Ingredients

- 2 cups brown quinoa, rinsed
- 6 tbsps plant-based yogurt
- 1 lime, juiced
- 4 tbsps chopped fresh cilantro
- 2 (5 oz) can black beans, drained
- 6 tbsps tomato salsa
- ½ avocado, sliced
- 4 radishes, shredded
- 2 tbsps pepitas (pumpkin seeds)

Directions

1. Cook the quinoa with 2 cups of slightly salted water in a medium pot over medium heat or until the liquid absorbs, 15 minutes.
2. Spoon the quinoa into serving bowls and fluff with a fork.
3. In a small bowl, mix the yogurt, lime juice, cilantro, and salt.

4. Divide this mixture on the quinoa and top with beans, salsa, avocado, radishes, and pepitas. Serve immediately.

Enjoy!!

LUNCH

Bulgur Wheat Salad

8 Servings

(Ready in about 25 minutes)

Nutrition: Calories: 359; Fat: 15.5g; Carbs: 48.1g; Protein: 10.1g

Ingredients

- 2 cups bulgur wheat
- 3 cups vegetable broth
- 2 teaspoons sea salt
- 2 teaspoons fresh ginger, minced
- 8 tablespoons olive oil
- 2 onions, chopped
- 16 ounces canned garbanzo beans, drained
- 4 large roasted peppers, sliced
- 4 tablespoons fresh parsley, roughly chopped

Directions

1. In a deep saucepan, bring the bulgur wheat and vegetable broth to a simmer; let it cook, covered, for 12 to 13 minutes.
2. Let it stand for about 10 minutes and fluff with a fork.

3. Add the remaining ingredients to the cooked bulgur wheat; serve at room temperature or well-chilled. Bon appétit!

Rice Pudding with Currants

8 Servings

(Ready in about 45 minutes)

Nutrition: Calories: 423; Fat: 5.3g; Carbs: 85g; Protein: 8.8g

Ingredients

- 3 cups water
- 2 cup white rice
- 5 cups oat milk, divided
- 1 cup white sugar
- A pinch of salt
- A pinch of grated nutmeg
- 2 teaspoons ground cinnamon
- 1 teaspoon vanilla extract
- 1 cup dried currants

Directions

1. In a saucepan, bring the water to a boil over medium-high heat. Immediately turn the heat to a simmer, add in the rice and let it cook for about 20 minutes.
2. Add in the milk, sugar, and spices and continue to cook for 20 minutes more, constantly stirring to prevent the rice from sticking to the pan.

3. Top with dried currants and serve at room temperature.

Bon appétit!

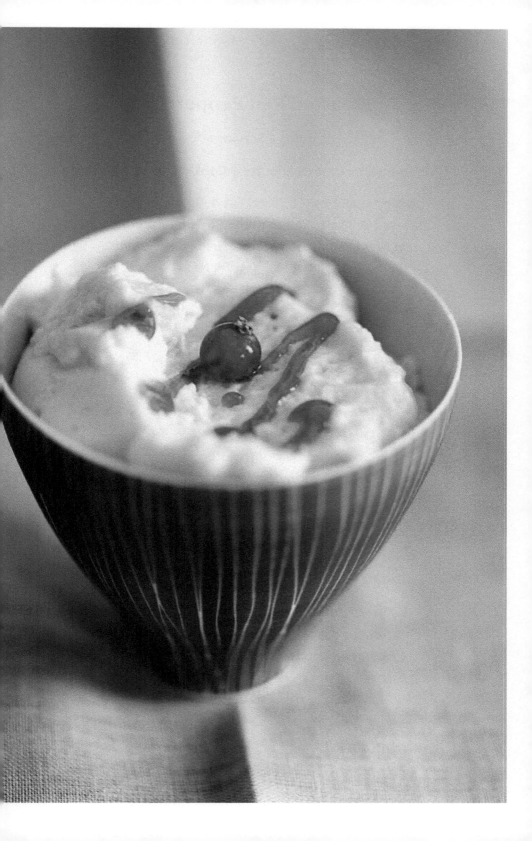

Roasted Red Pepper Pasta

4 Servings

Preparation Time: 5 minutes | **Cooking Time:** 05 minutes

Nutrition: Calories198, Total Fat 4. 9g, Saturated Fat 2. 2g, Cholesterol 31mg, Sodium 909mg, Total Carbohydrate 26. 8g, Dietary Fiber 1. 9g, Total Sugars 5. 6g, Protein 11. 9g

Ingredients:

- 4 cups vegetable broth
- 1 cup spaghetti
- 2 small onions
- 1 teaspoon garlic minced
- 1 cup roasted red peppers
- 1 cup roasted diced tomato
- 1/2 tablespoon dried mint
- 1/4 teaspoon crushed red pepper
- Freshly cracked black pepper
- 1 cup goat cheese

Directions:

1. In an Instant Pot, combine the vegetable broth, onion, garlic, red pepper slices, diced tomatoes, mint, crushed red pepper, and some freshly cracked black pepper. Stir these ingredients to combine. Add spaghetti to the Instant Pot.

2. Place lid on Instant Pot and lock into place to seal. Pressure Cook on High Pressure for 4 minutes. Use Quick Pressure Release.

3. Divide the goat cheese into tablespoon-sized pieces, then add them to the Instant Pot. Stir the pasta until the cheese melts in and creates a smooth sauce. Serve hot.

Pastalaya

4 Servings

Preparation Time: 5 minutes | **Cooking Time:** 05 minutes

Nutrition: Calories 351, Total Fat 6. 8g, Saturated Fat 3. 5g, Cholesterol 56mg. Sodium 869mg, Total Carbohydrate 45. 5g, Dietary Fiber 1. 5g, Total Sugars 2. 9g, Protein 26. 3g

Ingredients:

- 1 tablespoon avocado oil
- 1 teaspoon garlic powder
- 2 diced tomatoes
- ½ teaspoon dried basil
- ½ teaspoon smoked paprika
- ½ teaspoon dried rosemary
- Freshly cracked pepper
- 2 cups vegetable broth
- 1 cup of water
- 2 cups orzo pasta
- 2 tablespoons coconut cream
- 1 bunch fresh coriander

Directions:

1. In the Instant Pot, place the garlic powder and avocado oil, sauté for 15 seconds, or until the garlic is fragrant. Add diced tomatoes, basil, smoked paprika, rosemary, freshly cracked pepper, and orzo

pasta to the Instant Pot. Finally, add the vegetable broth and ½ cup of water, and stir until everything is evenly combined.

2. Place the lid on the Instant Pot, and bring the toggle switch into the "Sealing" position. Press Manual or Pressure Cook and adjust the time for 5 minutes.

3. When the five minutes are up, do a Natural-release for 5 minutes and then move the toggle switch to "Venting" to release the rest of the pressure in the pot.

4. Remove the lid. If the mixture looks watery, press "Sauté" and bring the mixture up to a boil and let it boil for a few minutes. It will thicken as it boils. Add the coconut cream and leek to the Instant Pot, stir and let warm through for a few minutes.

5. Serve and garnish with coriander toast.

Enjoy!

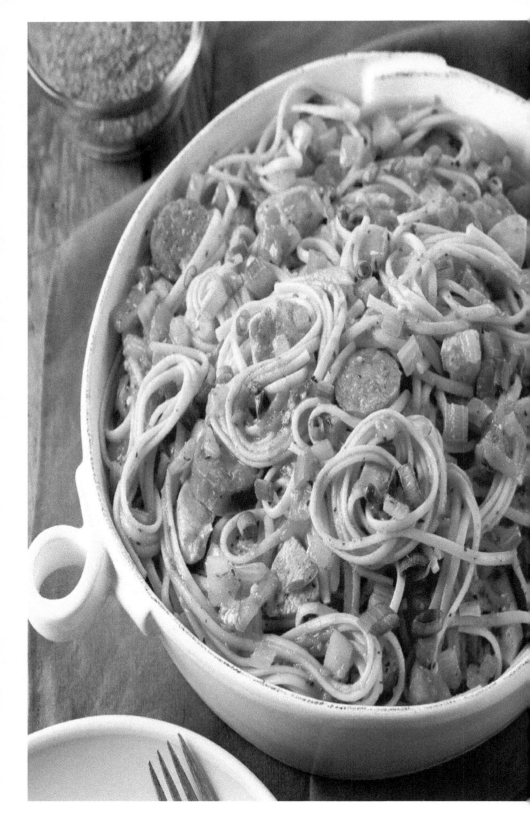

Corn and Chiles Fusilli

4 Servings

Preparation Time: 5 minutes | **Cooking Time:** 05 minutes

Nutrition: Calories 399, Total Fat 14. 4g, Saturated Fat 10g, Cholesterol 15mg, Sodium 531mg, Total Carbohydrate 56. 2g, Dietary Fiber 4. 9g, Total Sugars 7. 2g, Protein 15. 4g

Ingredients:

- 1 tablespoon butter
- 2 tablespoons garlic minced
- Salt and pepper to taste
- 4 oz. can green chills
- 1 cup frozen corn kernels
- ½ teaspoon cumin
- 1/4 teaspoon paprika
- 2 cups fusilli
- 2 cups vegetable broth
- ½ cup coconut cream
- 4 leeks, sliced
- 1/4 bunch parsley
- 2 oz. shredded mozzarella cheese

Directions:

1. In the Instant Pot, add butter when butter melt, place the minced garlic, salt, and pepper, then press Sauté on the Instant Pot.

2. Add the can of green chills (with juices), frozen corn kernels, cumin, and paprika.
3. Add the uncooked fusilli and vegetable broth to the Instant Pot.
4. Place the lid on the Instant Pot, and bring the toggle switch into the "Sealing" position. Press Manual or Pressure Cook and adjust the time for 5 minutes.
5. When the five minutes are up, do a Natural-release for 5 minutes and then move the toggle switch to "Venting" to release the rest of the pressure in the pot.
6. Remove the lid. If the mixture looks watery, press "Sauté," and bring the mixture up to a boil and let it boil for a few minutes. Then add the coconut cream and stir until it has fully coated the pasta. Stir in most of the sliced leek and parsley, reserving a little to sprinkle over the top, mozzarella on top of the pasta.

Creamy Pesto Pasta With Tofu & Broccoli

4 Servings

Preparation Time: 5 minutes | **Cooking Time:** 10 minutes

Nutrition: Calories 383, Total Fat 17. 8g, Saturated Fat 10. 1g, Cholesterol 39mg, Sodium 129mg, Total Carbohydrate 44g, Dietary Fiber 2. 4g, Total Sugars 3. 2g, Protein 13. 6g

Ingredients:

- 8 oz. Farfalle pasta
- 8 oz. frozen broccoli florets
- 1 tablespoon coconut oil
- 1 cup tofu
- ½ cup basil pesto
- ½ cup vegetable broth
- 4 oz. heavy cream

Directions:

1. In the Instant Pot, add Farfalline pasta, broccoli, coconut oil, tofu, basil pesto, vegetable broth. Cover the Instant Pot and lock it in.
2. Set the Manual or Pressure Cook timer for 10 minutes. Make sure the timer is set to "Sealing."
3. Once the timer reaches zero, quickly release the pressure. Add heavy cream.

Enjoy.

Green Avocado Carbonara

8 Servings

(Ready in 30 minutes)

Ingredients

- 16 tbsps flax seed powder
- 3 cups cashew cream cheese
- 11 tbsps psyllium husk powder
- 2 avocadoes, chopped
- 1 ¾ cups coconut cream
- Juice of ½ lemon
- 2 teaspoons onion powder
- 1 teaspoon garlic powder
- 1/2 cup olive oil
- Salt and black pepper to taste
- 1 cup grated plant-based Parmesan
- 8 tbsps toasted pecans

Directions

1. Preheat oven to 300 F.
2. In a medium bowl, mix the flax seed powder with 1 ½ cups water and allow sitting to thicken for 5 minutes.
3. Add the cashew cream cheese, salt, and psyllium husk powder.
4. Whisk until smooth batter forms.

5. Line a baking sheet with parchment paper, pour in the batter and cover with another parchment paper.
6. Use a rolling pin to flatten the dough into the sheet. Bake for 10-12 minutes.
7. Remove, take off the parchment papers and use a sharp knife to slice the pasta into thin strips lengthwise.
8. Cut each piece into halves, pour into a bowl, and set aside.
9. In a blender, combine avocado, coconut cream, lemon juice, onion powder, and garlic powder; puree until smooth.
10. Pour the olive oil over the pasta and stir to coat properly.
11. Pour the avocado sauce on top and mix.
12. Season with salt and black pepper.
13. Divide the pasta into serving plates, garnish with Parmesan cheese and pecans, and serve immediately.

Enjoy!

Curried Tofu with Buttery Cabbage

8 Servings
(Ready in 55 minutes)

Ingredients

- 4 cups tofu, cubed
- 2 tbsps + 3 ½ tbsp coconut oil
- 1 cup grated coconut
- 2 tsps yellow curry powder
- 1 tsp onion powder
- 4 cups Napa cabbage, grated
- 8 oz plant butter
- Salt and black pepper to taste
- Lemon wedges for serving

Directions

1. Drizzle 1 tablespoon of coconut oil on the tofu.
2. In a bowl, mix the shredded coconut, yellow curry powder, salt, and onion powder.
3. Toss the tofu cubes in the spice mixture.
4. Heat the remaining coconut oil in a non-stick skillet and fry the coated tofu until golden brown on all sides.
5. Transfer to a plate.
6. In another skillet, melt half of the plant butter, add, and sauté the cabbage until slightly caramelized. Then, season with salt and black pepper.

7. Dish the cabbage into serving plates with tofu and lemon wedges.
8. Melt the remaining plant butter in the skillet and drizzle over the cabbage and tofu. Serve.

Enjoy!

Mushroom Curry Pie

12 Servings

(Ready in 70 minutes)

Ingredients

Piecrust:

- 2 tbsps flax seed powder + 3 tbsp water
- 5/2 cups coconut flour
- 8 tbsps chia seeds
- 8 tbsps almond flour
- 2 tbsps psyllium husk powder
- 2 tsps baking powder
- 2 pinch of salt
- 6 tbsps olive oil
- 8 tbsps water

Filling:

- 2 cups chopped shiitake mushrooms
- 2 cups tofu mayonnaise
- 6 tbsps flax seed powder + 9 tbsp water
- 2 red bell peppers, finely chopped
- 2 tsps turmeric
- 1 tsp paprika
- 1 tsp garlic powder
- 1 cup cashew cream cheese
- 2 cups grated plant-based Parmesan

Directions

1. In two separate bowls, mix the different portions of flax seed powder with the respective quantity of water and set aside to absorb for 5 minutes.
2. Preheat oven to 350 F.
3. When the vegan "flax egg" is ready, pour the smaller quantity into a food processor, add in the pie crust ingredients and blend until a ball forms out of the dough.
4. Line a springform pan with parchment paper and grease with cooking spray.
5. Spread the dough on the bottom of the pan and bake for 15 minutes. In a bowl, add the remaining flax egg and all the filling ingredients, combine the mixture, and fill the piecrust.
6. Bake for 40 minutes.

Serve sliced.

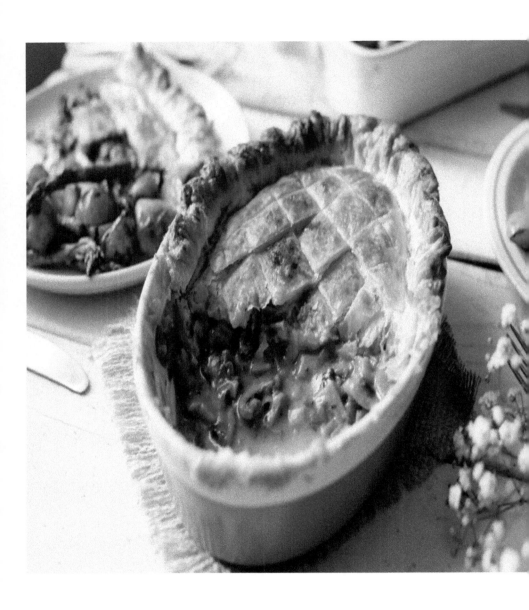

Cheesy Cauliflower Casserole

Ingredients

- 4 oz plant butter
- 2 white onions, finely chopped
- 1 cup celery stalks, finely chopped
- 2 green bell peppers, chopped
- Salt and black pepper to taste
- 2 small head cauliflowers, chopped
- 2 cups tofu mayonnaise
- 8 oz grated plant-based Parmesan
- 2 tsps red chili flakes

Directions

1. Preheat oven to 400 F.
2. Season onion, celery, and bell pepper with salt and black pepper.
3. In a bowl, mix cauliflower, tofu mayonnaise, Parmesan cheese, and red chili flakes.
4. Pour the mixture into a greased baking dish and add the vegetables; mix to distribute.
5. Bake for 20 minutes. Remove and serve warm.

DINNER

Picante Green Rice

8 Servings
(Ready in 35 minutes)

Ingredients

- 2 roasted bell pepper, chopped
- 6 small hot green chilies, chopped
- 5 cups vegetable broth
- 1 cup chopped fresh parsley
- 2 onions, chopped
- 4 garlic cloves, chopped
- Salt and black pepper to taste
- 1 tsp dried oregano
- 6 tbsps canola oil
- 2 cups long-grain brown rice
- 3 cups cooked black beans
- 4 tbsps minced fresh cilantro

Directions

1. In a food processor, place bell pepper, chilies, 1 cup of broth, parsley, onion, garlic, pepper, oregano, salt, and pepper, and blend until smooth.
2. Heat oil in a skillet over medium heat.
3. Add in rice and veggie mixture.
4. Cook for 5 minutes, stirring often.

5. Add in the remaining broth and bring to a boil, lower the heat, and simmer for 15 minutes.
6. Mix in beans and cook for another 5 minutes. Serve with cilantro.

Enjoy!

Bean & Pecan Sandwiches

8 Servings

(Ready in 20 minutes)

Ingredients

- 2 onions, chopped
- 2 garlic cloves, crushed
- 5/2 cups pecans, chopped
- 5/2 cups canned black beans
- 5/2 cups almond flour
- 4 tbsps minced fresh parsley
- 2 tbsps soy sauce
- 2 tsps Dijon mustard + to serve
- Salt and black pepper to taste
- 1 tsp ground sage
- 1 tsp sweet paprika
- 4 tbsps olive oil
- Bread slices
- Lettuce leaves and sliced tomatoes

Directions

1. Put the onion, garlic, and pecans in a blender and pulse until roughly ground.
2. Add in the beans and pulse until everything is well combined.

3. Transfer to a large mixing bowl and stir in the flour, parsley, soy sauce, mustard, salt, sage, paprika, and pepper.
4. Mold patties out of the mixture.
5. Heat the oil in a skillet over medium heat.
6. Brown the patties for 10 minutes on both sides.
7. To assemble, lay patties on the bread slices and top with mustard, lettuce, and tomato slices.

Enjoy!

Walnut Lentil Burgers

8 Servings

(Ready in 70 minutes)

Ingredients

- 4 tbsps olive oil

- 2 cups dry lentils, rinsed
- 4 carrots, grated
- 2 onions, diced
- 1 cup walnuts
- 2 tbsps tomato puree
- 5/2 cups almond flour
- 4 tsps curry powder
- 8 whole-grain buns

Directions

1. Place lentils in a pot and cover them with water. Bring to a boil and simmer for 15-20 minutes.
2. Meanwhile, combine the carrots, walnuts, onion, tomato puree, flour, curry powder, salt, and pepper in a bowl. Toss to coat. Once the lentils are ready, drain and transfer them into the veggie bowl.
3. Mash the mixture until sticky.
4. Shape the mixture into balls; flatten to make patties.

5. Heat the oil in a skillet over medium heat. Brown the patties for 8 minutes on both sides. To assemble, put the cakes on the buns and top with your desired toppings.

Enjoy!

Faro & Black Bean Loaf

12 Servings
(Ready in 50 minutes)

Ingredients

- 6 tbsps olive oil
- 2 onions, minced
- 2 cups faro
- 4 (15.5-oz) cans black beans, mashed
- 1 cup quick-cooking oats
- 1/6 cup whole-wheat flour
- 4 tbsps nutritional yeast
- 3 tsps dried thyme
- 1 tsp dried oregano

Directions

1. Heat the oil in a pot over medium heat.
2. Place in onion and sauté for 3 minutes.
3. Add in faro, 2 cups of water, salt, and pepper.
4. Bring to a boil, lower the heat and simmer for 20 minutes. Remove to a bowl.
5. Preheat oven to 350 F.
6. Add the mashed beans, oats, flour, yeast, thyme, and oregano to the faro bowl.
7. Toss to combine.

8. Taste and adjust the seasoning. Shape the mixture into a greased loaf. Bake for 20 minutes. Let cool for a few minutes. Slice and serve.

Sherry Shallot Beans

8 Servings
(Ready in 25 minutes)

Ingredients

- 4 tsps olive oil
- 8 shallots, chopped
- 2 tsps ground cumin
- 2 (14.5-oz) cans black beans
- 2 cups vegetable broth
- 4 tbsps sherry vinegar

Directions

1. Heat the oil in a pot over medium heat.
2. Place in shallots and cumin and cook for 3 minutes until soft.
3. Stir in beans and broth.
4. Bring to a boil, then lower the heat and simmer for 10 minutes.
5. Add in sherry vinegar, increase the heat and cook for an additional 3 minutes. Serve warm.

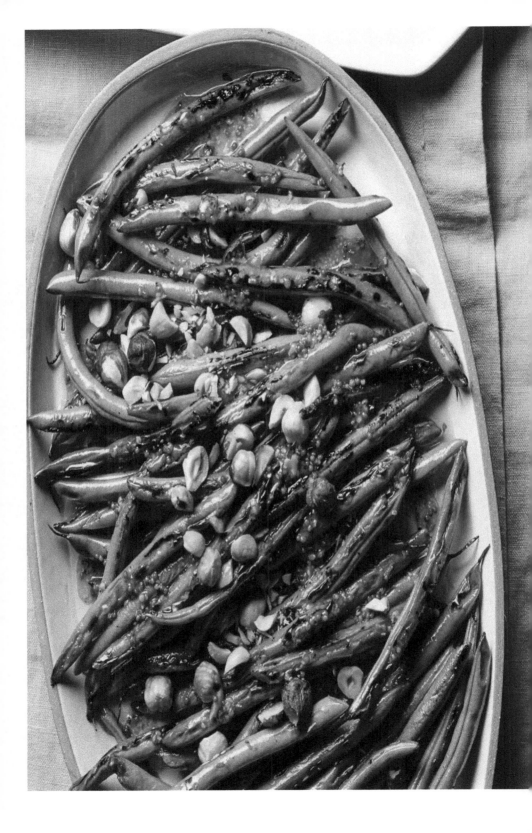

Celery Buckwheat Croquettes

24 Servings
(Ready in 25 minutes)

Ingredients

- 5 cups cooked buckwheat groats
- 2 cups cooked brown rice
- 12 tbsps olive oil
- 1 cup minced onion
- 4 celeries stalk, chopped
- 1 cup shredded carrots
- 1/3 cup whole-wheat flour
- 1 cup chopped fresh parsley
- Salt and black pepper to taste

Directions

1. Combine the groats and rice in a bowl. Set aside. Heat 1 tbsp of oil in a skillet over medium heat. Place in onion, celery, and carrot and cook for 5 minutes. Transfer to the rice bowl.
2. Mix in flour, parsley, salt, and pepper.
3. Place in the fridge for 20 minutes.
4. Mold the mixture into cylinder-shaped balls. Heat the remaining oil in a skillet over medium heat. Fry the croquettes for 8 minutes, occasionally turning until golden.

Rich Bulgur Salad with Herbs

8 Servings

(Ready in about 20 minutes + chilling time)

Nutrition: Calories: 408; Fat: 18.3g; Carbs: 51.8g; Protein: 13.1g

Ingredients

- 4 cups water
- 2 cups bulgur
- 24 ounces canned chickpeas, drained
- 2 Persian cucumbers, thinly sliced
- 4 bell peppers, seeded and thinly sliced
- 2 jalapeno peppers, seeded and thinly sliced
- 4 Roma tomatoes, sliced
- 2 onions, thinly sliced
- 4 tablespoons fresh basil, chopped
- 4 tablespoons fresh parsley, chopped
- 4 tablespoons fresh mint, chopped
- 4 tablespoons fresh chives, chopped
- 8 tablespoons olive oil
- 2 tablespoons balsamic vinegar
- 2 tablespoons lemon juice
- 2 teaspoons fresh garlic, pressed
- Sea salt and freshly ground black pepper, to taste
- 4 tablespoons nutritional yeast
- 1 cup Kalamata olives, sliced

Directions

1. In a saucepan, bring the water and bulgur to a boil. Immediately turn the heat to a simmer and let it cook for about 20 minutes or until the bulgur is tender and water is almost absorbed. Fluff with a fork and spread on a large tray to let cool.
2. Place the bulgur in a salad bowl followed by the chickpeas, cucumber, peppers, tomatoes, onion, basil, parsley, mint, and chives.
3. In a small mixing dish, whisk the olive oil, balsamic vinegar, lemon juice, garlic, salt, and black pepper. Dress the salad and toss to combine.
4. Sprinkle nutritional yeast over the top, garnish with olives and serve at room temperature. Bon appétit!

Authentic Italian Panzanella Salad

3 Servings

Nutrition: Calories: 334; Fat: 20.4g; Carbs: 33.3g; Protein: 8.3g

Ingredients

- 6 cups artisan bread, broken into 1-inch cubes
- 3/2-pounds asparagus, trimmed and cut into bite-sized pieces
- 8 tablespoons extra-virgin olive oil
- 2 red onions, chopped
- 4 tablespoons fresh lime juice
- 2 teaspoons deli mustard
- 4 medium heirloom tomatoes, diced
- 4 cups arugula
- 4 cups baby spinach
- 4 Italian peppers, seeded and sliced
- Sea salt and ground black pepper, to taste

Directions

1. Arrange the bread cubes on a parchment-lined baking sheet. Bake in the preheated oven at 310 degrees F for about 20 minutes, rotating the baking sheet twice during the baking time; reserve.
2. Turn the oven to 420 degrees F and toss the asparagus with 1 tablespoon of olive oil. Roast the

asparagus for about 15 minutes or until crisp-tender.

3. Toss the remaining ingredients in a salad bowl; top with the roasted asparagus and toasted bread.

Bon appétit!

Cannellini Bean Soup with Kale

10 Servings

(Ready in about 25 minutes)

Nutrition: Calories: 188; Fat: 4.7g; Carbs: 24.5g; Protein: 11.1g

Ingredients

- 2 tablespoons olive oil
- 1 teaspoon ginger, minced
- 1 teaspoon cumin seeds
- 2 red onions, chopped
- 2 carrots, trimmed and chopped
- 2 parsnips, trimmed and chopped
- 4 garlic cloves, minced
- 10 cups vegetable broth
- 24 ounces Cannellini beans, drained
- 4 cups kale, torn into pieces
- Sea salt and ground black pepper, to taste

Directions

1. In a heavy-bottomed pot, heat the olive over medium-high heat. Now, sauté the ginger and cumin for 1 minute or so.

2. Now, add in the onion, carrot, and parsnip; continue sautéing an additional 3 minutes or until the vegetables are just tender.
3. Add in the garlic and continue to sauté for 1 minute or until aromatic.
4. Then, pour in the vegetable broth and bring it to a boil. Immediately reduce the heat to a simmer and let it cook for 10 minutes.
5. Fold in the Cannellini beans and kale; continue to simmer until the kale wilts and everything is thoroughly heated. Season with salt and pepper to taste.
6. Ladle into individual bowls and serve hot.
   Bon appétit!

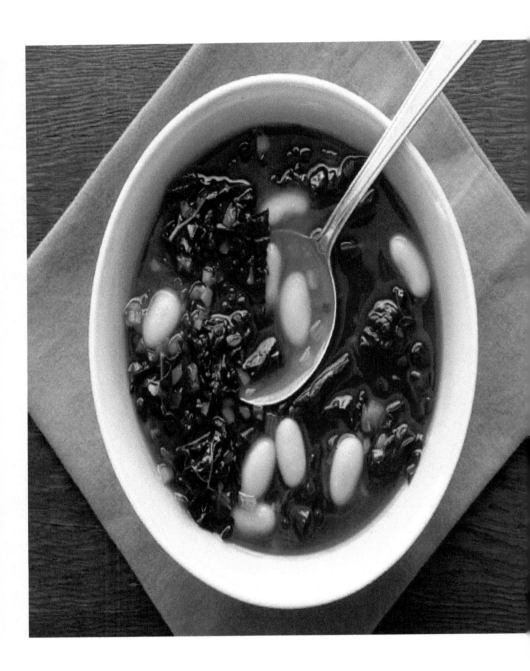

Roasted Asparagus and Avocado Salad

4 Servings

(Ready in about 20 minutes + chilling time)

Nutrition: Calories: 378; Fat: 33.2g; Carbs: 18.6g; Protein: 7.8g

Ingredients

- 2-pounds asparagus, trimmed, cut into bite-sized pieces
- 2 white onions, chopped
- 4 garlic cloves, minced
- 2 Roma tomatoes, sliced
- 1/2 cup olive oil
- 1/2 cup balsamic vinegar
- 2 tablespoons stone-ground mustard
- 4 tablespoons fresh parsley, chopped
- 2 tablespoons fresh cilantro, chopped
- 2 tablespoons fresh basil, chopped
- Sea salt and ground black pepper, to taste
- 2 small avocados, pitted and diced
- 1 cup pine nuts, roughly chopped

Directions

1. Begin by preheating your oven to 420 degrees F.

2. Toss the asparagus with 1 tablespoon of the olive oil and arrange them on a parchment-lined roasting pan.
3. Bake for about 15 minutes, rotating the pan once or twice to promote even cooking. Let it cool completely and place it in your salad bowl.
4. Toss the asparagus with the vegetables, olive oil, vinegar, mustard, and herbs. Salt and pepper to taste.
5. Toss to combine and top with avocado and pine nuts.

Bon appétit!

DESSERTS

Strawberry Coconut Ice Cream

4 Servings

Preparation Time: 5 minutes

Nutrition: Calories: 100 Cal, Fat: 100 g, Carbs: 100g. Protein: 100 g, Fiber: 100 g

Ingredients:

- 4 cups frozen strawberries
- 1 vanilla bean, seeded
- 28 ounces coconut cream
- 1/2 cup maple syrup

Directions:

1. Place cream in a food processor and pulse for 1 minute until soft peaks come together.
2. Then tip the cream in a bowl, add remaining ingredients into the blender and blend until a thick mixture comes together.
3. Add the mixture into the cream, fold until combined, and then transfer ice cream into a freezer-safe bowl and freeze for 4 hours until firm, whisking every 20 minutes after 1 hour.
   Serve straight away.

Rainbow Fruit Salad

8 Servings

Preparation Time: 10 minutes

Nutrition: Calories: 88.1 Cal Fat: 0.4 g Carbs: 22.6 g Protein: 1.1 g Fiber: 2.8 g

Ingredients:

For the Fruit Salad:

- 2 pounds strawberries, hulled, sliced
- 2 cups kiwis, halved, cubed
- 2 1/4 cups blueberries
- 2 1/3 cups blackberries
- 2 cups pineapple chunks

For the Maple Lime Dressing:

- 4 teaspoons lime zest
- ½ cup maple syrup
- 2 tablespoons lime juice

Directions:

1. Prepare the salad, and for this, take a bowl, place all its ingredients and toss until mixed.
2. Prepare the dressing, and for this, take a small bowl, place all its ingredients and whisk well.
3. Drizzle the dressing over salad, toss until coated, and serve.

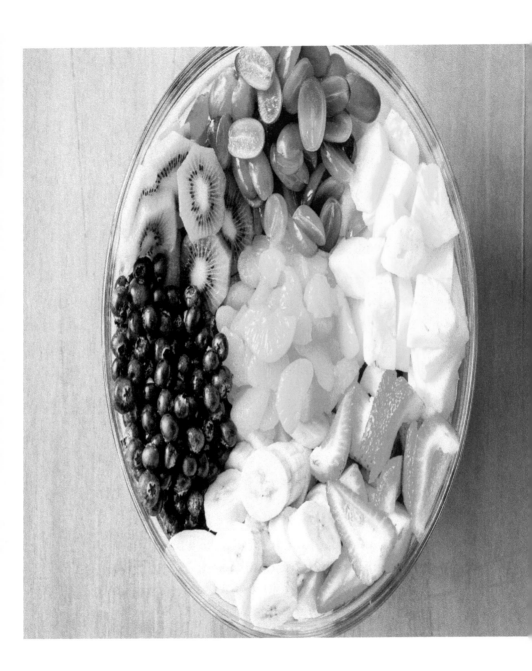

Apple Raspberry Cobbler

8 Servings

Preparation Time: 15-30 minutes | **Cooking Time:**50 minutes

Nutrition: Calories 539 Fats 12g Carbs 105. 7g Protein 8. 2g

Ingredients:

- 6 apples, peeled, cored, and chopped
- 4 tbsps pure date sugar
- 2 cups fresh raspberries
- 4 tbsps unsalted plant butter
- 1 cup whole-wheat flour
- 2 cups toasted rolled oats
- 4 tbsps pure date sugar
- 2 tsps cinnamon powder

Directions:

1. Preheat the oven to 350 F and grease a baking dish with some plant butter.
2. Add the apples, date sugar, and 3 tbsp of water to a medium pot. Cook over low heat until the date sugar melts, and then mix in the raspberries. Cook until the fruits soften, 10 minutes.
3. Pour and spread the fruit mixture into the baking dish and set aside.

4. In a blender, add the plant butter, flour, oats, date sugar, and cinnamon powder. Pulse a few times until crumbly.
5. Spoon and spread the mixture on the fruit mix until evenly layered.
6. Bake in the oven for 25 to 30 minutes or until golden brown on top.
7. Remove the dessert, allow cooling for 2 minutes, and serve.

Aunt´s Apricot Tarte Tatin

8 Servings

(Ready in 20 minutes)

Ingredients

- 8 tbsps flaxseed powder
- 1/2 cup almond flour
- 6 tbsps whole-wheat flour
- 1 tsp salt
- 1/2 cup cold plant butter, crumbled
- 6 tbsps pure maple syrup
- 8 tbsps melted plant butter
- 6 tsps pure maple syrup
- 2 tsps vanilla extract
- 2 lemons, juiced
- 24 apricots, halved and pitted
- 1 cup coconut cream
- 8 fresh basil leaves

Directions

1. Preheat the oven to 350 F and grease a large pie pan with cooking spray.
2. In a medium bowl, mix the flaxseed powder with 12 tbsp water and allow thickening for 5 minutes.
3. In a large bowl, combine the flour and salt. Add the plant butter, and using an electric hand mixer, whisk until crumbly. Pour in the vegan "flax egg" and

maple syrup and mix until smooth dough forms. Flatten the dough on a flat surface, cover with plastic wrap, and refrigerate for 1 hour.

4. Dust a working surface with almond flour, remove the dough onto the surface, and using a rolling pin, flatten the dough into a 1-inch diameter circle. Set aside. In a large bowl, mix the plant butter, maple syrup, vanilla, and lemon juice. Add the apricots to the mixture and coat well.

5. Arrange the apricots (open side down) in the pie pan and lay the dough on top. Press to fit and cut off the dough hanging on the edges. Brush the top with more plant butter and bake in the oven for 35 to 40 minutes or until golden brown and puffed up.

6. Remove the pie pan from the oven, allow cooling for 5 minutes, and run a butter knife around the edges of the pastry. Invert the dessert onto a large plate, spread the coconut cream on top, and garnish with the basil leaves. Slice and serve.

Vegan Cheesecake with Blueberries

12 Servings

(Ready in 1 hour 30 minutes + chilling time)

Ingredients

- 4 oz plant butter

- 2 ¼ cups almond flour
- 6 tbsps Swerve sugar
- 2 tsps vanilla extract
- 6 tbsps flaxseed powder
- 4 cups cashew cream cheese
- 1 cup coconut cream
- 2 tsps lemon zest
- 4 oz fresh blueberries

Directions

1. Preheat oven to 350 F and grease a springform pan with cooking spray. Line with parchment paper.

2. To make the crust, melt the plant butter in a skillet over low heat until nutty in flavor. Turn the heat off and stir in almond flour, 2 tbsp of Swerve sugar, and half of the vanilla until a dough forms. Press the mixture into the springform pan and bake for 8 minutes.

3. Mix flaxseed powder with 9 tbsp water and allow sitting for 5 minutes to thicken. In a bowl, combine

cashew cream cheese, coconut cream, remaining Swerve sugar, lemon zest, remaining vanilla extract, and vegan "flax egg."

4. Remove the crust from the oven and pour the mixture on top. Use a spatula to layer evenly.
5. Bake the cake for 15 minutes at 400 F. Then, reduce the heat to 230 F and bake for 45-60 minutes. Remove to cool completely.
6. Refrigerate overnight and scatter the blueberries on top. Serve.

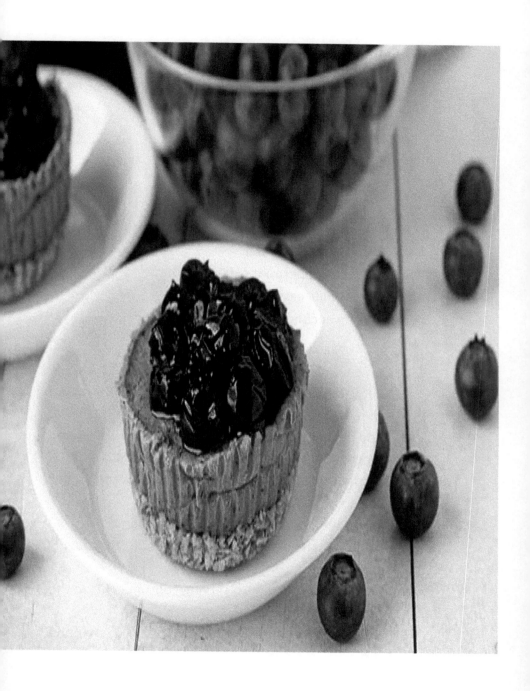

Chocolate Peppermint Mousse

8 Servings

(Ready in 10 minutes)

Ingredients

- 1/2 cup Swerve sugar, divided
- 8 oz cashew cream cheese, softened
- 6 tbsps cocoa powder
- 5/2 tsps peppermint extract
- 1 tsp vanilla extract
- 1/6 cup coconut cream

Directions

1. Put 2 tablespoons of Swerve sugar, cashew cream cheese, and cocoa powder in a blender.
2. Add the peppermint extract, ¼ cup warm water, and process until smooth. In a bowl, whip vanilla extract, coconut cream, and the remaining Swerve sugar using a whisk.
3. Fetch out 5-6 tablespoons for garnishing.
4. Fold in the cocoa mixture until thoroughly combined.
5. Spoon the mousse into serving cups and chill in the fridge for 30 minutes.
6. Garnish with the reserved whipped cream and serve.

Indian-Style Hummus Dip

20 Servings

(Ready in about 10 minutes)

Nutrition: Calories: 171; Fat: 10.4g; Carbs: 15.3g; Protein: 5.4g

Ingredients

- 40 ounces canned or boiled chickpeas, drained
- 2 teaspoons garlic, sliced
- 1/2 cup tahini
- 1/2 cup olive oil
- 2 limes, freshly squeezed
- 1/2 teaspoon turmeric
- 1 teaspoon cumin powder
- 2 teaspoons curry powder
- 2 teaspoons coriander seeds
- 1/2 cup chickpea liquid, or more, as needed
- 4 tablespoons fresh cilantro, roughly chopped

Directions

1. Blitz the chickpeas, garlic, tahini, olive oil, lime, turmeric, cumin, curry powder, and coriander seeds in your blender or food processor.

2. Blend until your desired consistency is reached, gradually adding the chickpea liquid.
3. Place in your refrigerator until ready to serve. Garnish with fresh cilantro.
4. Serve with naan bread or veggie sticks, if desired. Bon appétit!

Mexican-Style Onion Rings

12 Servings

(Ready in about 35 minutes)

Nutrition: Calories: 213; Fat: 10.6g; Carbs: 26.2g; Protein: 4.3g

Ingredients

- 4 medium onions, cut into rings
- 1/2 cup all-purpose flour
- 1/2 cup spelt flour
- 1/6 cup rice milk, unsweetened
- 1/6 cup ale beer
- Sea salt and ground black pepper, to season
- 1 teaspoon cayenne pepper
- 1 teaspoon mustard seeds
- 2 cups tortilla chips, crushed
- 2 tablespoons olive oil

Directions

1. Start by preheating your oven to 420 degrees F.
2. In a shallow bowl, mix the flour, milk, and beer.
3. In another shallow bowl, mix the spices with the crushed tortilla chips. Dredge the onion rings in the flour mixture.

4. Then, roll them over the spiced mixture, pressing down to coat well.
5. Arrange the onion rings on a parchment-lined baking pan. Brush them with olive oil and bake for approximately 30 minutes.

Bon appétit!

Cucumber Rounds with Hummus

12 Servings

(Ready in about 10 minutes)

Nutrition: Calories: 88; Fat: 3.6g; Carbs: 11.3g; Protein: 2.6g

Ingredients

- 2 cups hummus, preferably homemade
- 4 large tomatoes, diced
- 1 teaspoon red pepper flakes
- Sea salt and ground black pepper, to taste
- 4 English cucumbers, sliced into rounds

Directions

1. Divide the hummus dip between the cucumber rounds.
2. Top them with tomatoes; sprinkle red pepper flakes, salt, and black pepper over each cucumber.
3. Serve well chilled, and enjoy!

Spinach, Chickpea and Garlic Crostini

6 Servings

(Ready in about 10 minutes)

Nutrition: Calories: 242; Fat: 6.1g; Carbs: 38.5g; Protein: 8.9g

Ingredients

- 2 baguettes, cut into slices
- 8 tablespoons extra-virgin olive oil
- Sea salt and red pepper, to season
- 6 garlic cloves, minced
- 2 cups boiled chickpeas, drained
- 4 cups spinach
- 2 tablespoons fresh lemon juice

Directions

1. Preheat your broiler.
2. Brush the slices of bread with 2 tablespoons of the olive oil and sprinkle with sea salt and red pepper. Place under the preheated broiler for about 2 minutes or until lightly toasted.
3. In a mixing bowl, thoroughly combine the garlic, chickpeas, spinach, lemon juice, and the remaining 2 tablespoons of the olive oil.
4. Spoon the chickpea mixture onto each toast.

Bon appétit!

SNACKS

Roasted Pepper and Tomato Dip

20 Servings

(Ready in about 35 minutes)

Nutrition: Calories: 90; Fat: 5.7g; Carbs: 8.5g; Protein: 1.9g

Ingredients

- 8 red bell peppers
- 8 tomatoes
- 8 tablespoons olive oil
- 2 red onions, chopped
- 8 garlic cloves
- 8 ounces canned garbanzo beans, drained
- Sea salt and ground black pepper, to taste

Directions

1. Start by preheating your oven to 400 degrees F.
2. Place the peppers and tomatoes on a parchment-lined baking pan. Bake for about 30 minutes; peel the peppers and transfer them to your food processor along with the roasted tomatoes.
3. Meanwhile, heat 2 tablespoons of the olive oil in a frying pan over medium-high heat. Sauté the onion and garlic for about 5 minutes or until they've softened.

4. Add the sautéed vegetables to your food processor. Add in the garbanzo beans, salt, pepper, and the remaining olive oil; process until creamy and smooth.

Bon appétit!

Classic Party Mix

15 Servings

(Ready in about 1 hour 5 minutes)

Nutrition: Calories: 290; Fat: 12.2g; Carbs: 39g; Protein: 7.5g

Ingredients

- 10 cups vegan corn cereal
- 6 cups vegan mini pretzels
- 2 cups almonds, roasted
- 1 cup pepitas, toasted
- 2 tablespoons nutritional yeast
- 2 tablespoons balsamic vinegar
- 2 tablespoons soy sauce
- 2 teaspoons garlic powder
- 1/6 cup vegan butter

Directions

1. Start by preheating your oven to 250 degrees F. Line a large baking pan with parchment paper or a Silpat mat.
2. Mix the cereal, pretzels, almonds, and pepitas in a serving bowl.
3. In a small saucepan, melt the remaining ingredients over moderate heat. Pour the sauce over the cereal/nut mixture.

4. Bake for about 1 hour, stirring every 15 minutes, until golden and fragrant. Transfer it to a wire rack to cool completely.

Bon appétit!

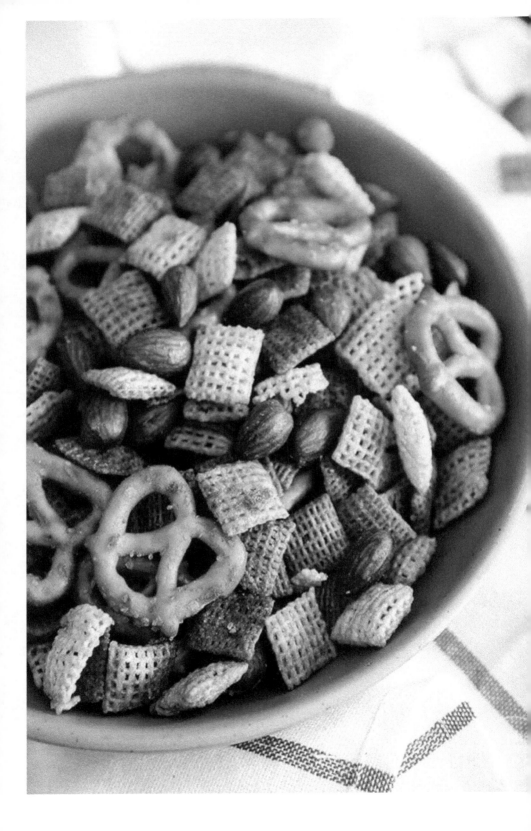

Olive Oil Garlic Crostini

8 Servings

(Ready in about 10 minutes)

Nutrition: Calories: 289; Fat: 8.2g; Carbs: 44.9g; Protein: 9.5g

Ingredients

- 2 whole-grain baguettes, sliced
- 8 tablespoons extra-virgin olive oil
- 1 teaspoon sea salt
- 6 cloves of garlic, halved

Directions

1. Preheat your broiler.
2. Brush each slice of bread with the olive oil and sprinkle with sea salt. Place under the preheated broiler for about 2 minutes or until lightly toasted.
3. Rub each slice of bread with the garlic and serve. Bon appétit!

Vegetarian Irish Stew

6 Servings

Preparation Time: 5 minutes | **Cooking Time:** 38 minutes

Nutrition: Calories: 117.4 Cal Fat: 4 g Carbs: 22.8 g Protein: 6.5 g Fiber: 7.3 g

Ingredients:

- 2 cups textured vegetable protein, chunks
- 1 cup split red lentils
- 4 medium onions, peeled, sliced
- 2 cups sliced parsnip
- 4 cups sliced mushrooms
- 2 cups diced celery,
- 1/2 cup flour
- 8 cups vegetable stock
- 2 cups rutabaga
- 2 bay leaves
- 1 cup fresh parsley
- 2 teaspoons sugar
- 1/2 teaspoon ground black pepper
- 1/2 cup soy sauce
- 1/2 teaspoon thyme
- 4 teaspoons marmite
- 1/2 teaspoon rosemary
- 1/3 teaspoon salt
- 1/2 teaspoon marjoram

Directions:

1. Take a large soup pot, place it over medium heat, add oil and when it gets hot, add onions and cook for 5 minutes until softened.
2. Then switch heat to the low level, sprinkle with flour, stir well, add remaining ingredients, stir until combined, and simmer for 30 minutes until vegetables have cooked.
3. When done, season the stew with salt and black pepper and then serve.

Spinach and Cannellini Bean Stew

12 Servings

Preparation Time: 10 minutes | **Cooking Time:** 15 minutes

Nutrition: Calories: 242 Cal Fat: 10.2 g Carbs: 31 g Protein: 11 g Fiber: 8.5 g

Ingredients:

- 56 ounces cooked cannellini beans
- 48 ounces tomato passata
- 34 ounces spinach chopped
- ½ teaspoon ground black pepper
- 1/3 teaspoon salt
- 2 ¼ teaspoon curry powder
- 2 cups cashew butter
- ¼ teaspoon cardamom
- 4 tablespoons olive oil
- 2 teaspoons salt
- 1 cup cashews
- 4 tablespoons chopped basil
- 4 tablespoons chopped parsley

Directions:

1. Take a large saucepan, place it over medium heat, add 1 tablespoon oil and when hot, add spinach and cook for 3 minutes until fried.
2. Then stir in butter and tomato passata until well mixed, bring the mixture to a near boil, add beans,

and season with ¼ teaspoon curry powder, black pepper, and salt.

3. Take a small saucepan, place it over medium heat, add remaining oil, stir in cashew, stir in salt and curry powder and cook for 4 minutes until toasted, set aside until required.

4. Transfer cooked stew into a bowl, top with roasted cashews, basil, and parsley, and then serve.

Brussel Sprouts Stew

4 Servings

Preparation Time: 10 minutes | **Cooking Time:** 55 minutes

Nutrition: Calories: 156 Cal Fat: 3 g Carbs: 22 g Protein: 12 g Fiber: 5.1100 g

Ingredients:

- 35 ounces Brussels sprouts
- 10 medium potatoes, peeled, chopped
- 2 medium onions, peeled, chopped
- 4 carrots, peeled, cubed
- 4 teaspoons smoked paprika
- 1/4 teaspoon ground black pepper
- 1/4 teaspoon salt
- 6 tablespoons caraway seeds
- 1 teaspoon red chili powder
- 2 tablespoons nutmeg
- 2 tablespoons olive oil
- 7 cups hot vegetable stock

Directions:

1. Take a large pot, place it over medium-high heat, add oil, and when hot, add onion and cook for 1 minute.
2. Then add carrot and potato, cook for 2 minutes, then add Brussel sprouts and cook for 5 minutes.
3. Stir in all the spices, pour in vegetable stock, bring the mixture to boil, switch heat to medium-low and

simmer for 45 minutes until cooked and stew reaches the desired thickness.

Serve straight away.

Vegetarian Gumbo

8 Servings

Preparation Time: 10 minutes | **Cooking Time:** 45 minutes

Nutrition: Calories: 160 Cal Fat: 7.3 g Carbs: 20 g Protein: 7 g Fiber: 5.7 g

Ingredients:

- 3 cups diced zucchini
- 16-ounces cooked red beans
- 8 cups sliced okra
- 3 cups diced green pepper
- 3 cups chopped white onion
- 3 cups diced red bell pepper
- 16 cremini mushrooms, quartered
- 2 cups sliced celery
- 6 teaspoons minced garlic
- 2 medium tomatoes, chopped
- 2 teaspoons red pepper flakes
- 2 teaspoons dried thyme
- 6 tablespoons all-purpose flour
- 2 tablespoons smoked paprika
- 2 teaspoons dried oregano
- 1/2 teaspoon nutmeg
- 2 teaspoons soy sauce
- 3 teaspoons liquid smoke
- 4 tablespoons mustard

- 2 tablespoons apple cider vinegar
- 2 tablespoons Worcestershire sauce, vegetarian
- 1 teaspoon hot sauce
- 6 tablespoons olive oil
- 8 cups vegetable stock
- 1 cup sliced green onion
- 8 cups cooked jasmine rice

Directions:

1. Take a Dutch oven, place it over medium heat, add oil and flour and cook for 5 minutes until fragrant.
2. Switch heat to the medium low level, and continue cooking for 20 minutes until the roux becomes dark brown, whisking constantly.
3. Meanwhile, place the tomato in a food processor, add garlic and onion along with remaining ingredients, except for stock, zucchini, celery, mushroom, green and red bell pepper, and pulse for 2 minutes until smooth.
4. Pour the mixture into the pan, return pan over medium-high heat, stir until mixed, and cook for 5 minutes until all the liquid has evaporated.
5. Stir in stock, bring it to simmer, then add remaining vegetables and simmer for 20 minutes until tender.
6. Garnish gumbo with green onions and serve with rice.

Mushroom Broccoli Faux Risotto

4 Servings

(Ready in 25 minutes)

Ingredients

- 8 oz plant butter
- 2 cups cremini mushrooms, chopped
- 4 garlic cloves, minced
- 2 small red onions, finely chopped
- 2 large head broccolis, grated
- 5/2 cups white wine
- 2 cups coconut whipping cream
- 5/2 cups grated plant-based Parmesan
- Freshly chopped thyme

Directions

1. Place a pot over medium heat, add, and melt the plant butter. Sauté the mushrooms in the pot until golden, about 5 minutes. Add the garlic and onions and cook for 3 minutes or until fragrant and soft. Mix in the broccoli, 1 cup water, and half of the white wine. Season with salt and black pepper and simmer the ingredients (uncovered) for 8 to 10 minutes or until the broccoli is soft.

2. Mix in the coconut whipping cream and simmer until most of the cream has evaporated. Turn the heat off and stir in the parmesan cheese and thyme until well incorporated. Dish the risotto and serve warm or with grilled tofu.

Mixed Seed Crackers

6 Servings

(Ready in 57 minutes)

Ingredients

- 1/6 cup sesame seed flour
- 1/6 cup pumpkin seeds
- 1/6 cup sunflower seeds
- 1/6 cup sesame seeds
- 1/6 cup chia seeds
- 2 tbsps psyllium husk powder
- 2 tsps salt
- 1/2 cup plant butter, melted
- 2 cups boiling water

Directions

1. Preheat oven to 300 F.

2. Combine the sesame seed flour with the pumpkin seeds, sunflower seeds, sesame seeds, chia seeds, psyllium husk powder, and salt. Pour in the plant butter and hot water and mix the ingredients until a dough forms with a gel-like consistency.

3. Line a baking sheet with parchment paper and place the dough on the sheet. Cover the dough with another parchment paper and, with a rolling pin, flatten the dough into the baking sheet. Remove the parchment paper on top.

4. Tuck the baking sheet in the oven and bake for 45 minutes. Allow the crackers to cool and dry in the oven, about 10 minutes. After, remove the sheet and break the crackers into small pieces. Serve.

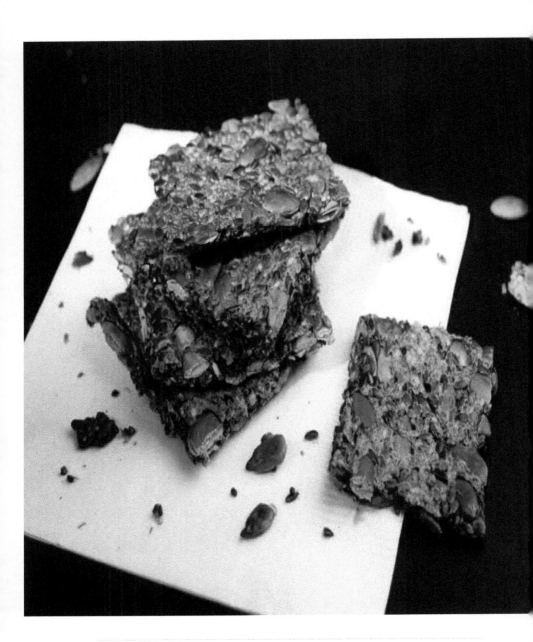

Spinach Chips with Guacamole Hummus

8 Servings

(Ready in 20 minutes)

Ingredients

- 1 cup baby spinach
- 2 tbsps olive oil
- 1 tsp plain vinegar
- 6 large avocados, chopped
- 1 cup chopped parsley + for garnish
- 1 cup melted plant butter
- 1/2 cup pumpkin seeds
- 1/2 cup sesame paste
- Juice from 1 lemon
- 2 garlic cloves, minced
- 1 tsp coriander powder
- Salt and black pepper to taste

Directions

1. Preheat oven to 300 F. Put spinach in a bowl and toss with olive oil, vinegar, and salt. Place in a parchment paper-lined baking sheet and bake until the leaves are crispy but not burned, about 15 minutes.

2. Place avocado into the bowl of a food processor. Add in parsley, plant butter, pumpkin seeds, sesame

paste, lemon juice, garlic, coriander powder, salt, and black pepper. Puree until smooth. Spoon the hummus into a bowl and garnish with parsley. Serve with spinach chips.

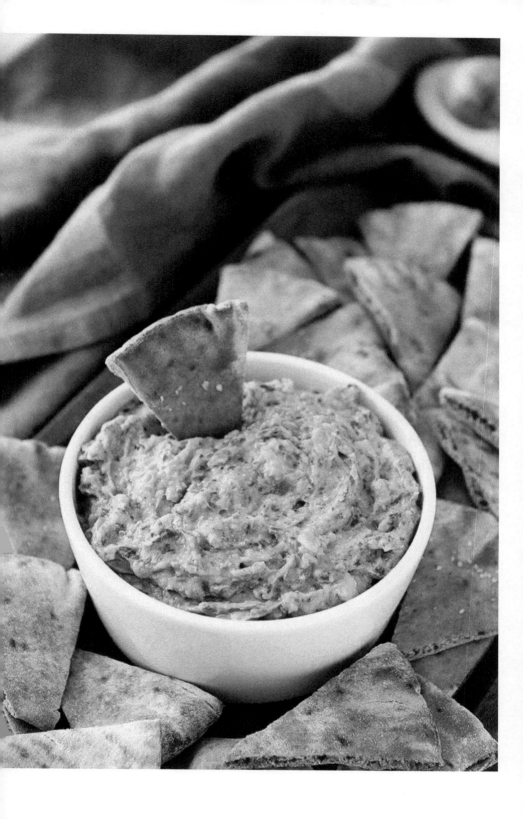

CONCLUSION

There are a plethora of compelling reasons to make a positive difference and transition to a plant-based diet. A plant-based diet will increase your quality of life by providing you with more energy and stamina, assisting you in losing excess body weight, and perhaps even extending your time on this magnificent world. Too much energy and fossil fuels are lost in the process of obtaining meat and other animal products, shipping them over miles and miles of road, and refining them. You will also be bringing a genuine and important difference to the future of our planet Earth by making the transition.

By switching to rich plant-based meals, we can save the earth and also take care of ourselves.

Thank you for taking time to read this.

Lightning Source UK Ltd.
Milton Keynes UK
UKHW052220060421
381512UK00001BA/37